This book is dedicated to the yoga teachers who move mountains to share their passion with the world.

Acknowledgments

This book would not exist without the help of a community of people. My thanks must first go to Steve Haase who helped and cheered me on from the start and by now has read this book more than I have.

Thank you to all of my inspiring friends on the path who became involved with this project and provided so much insight and love. Special Thanks to Julie & John Aquin, Julie Trafford, Jeff Carreira, Brian Hunt, Donna Powell, Katie McClelland Kate Connell, Jenny Ravikumar, Brittany Mills and Amy Jo Gengler.

Finally, I want to thank the teachers who opened up to me. Without your trust and the questions you asked, I would never have dreamed of sharing my experiences. I hope this book helps to change your life.

Introduction

Welcome to the A-Z of being a Successful Yoga Teacher. This book is meant to help you identify the key ingredients you need to be a powerful and engaging yoga instructor. Teaching yoga is not just about showing up to class to deliver your thoughts, philosophy and knowledge about the practice, it's about helping people live healthier and richer lives.

In order to make a successful living as a teacher (yes it is possible) you must be an entrepreneur, a marketer, and a powerful instructor while living a life that others aspire to. Think of that ever-popular yoga teacher phrase, "Walk your talk."

In the pages to come we will dive in to the A-Z of Being a Successful Yoga Teacher, touching upon all aspects of what it takes to maintain your energy, your business and your sanity as you master the different roles involved. In order to help you stay on track, process your thoughts, and get support from other teachers, I invite you to join the exclusive (and free) Facebook community <u>Being a Successful Yoga Teacher</u>.

Let's dive in!

CHAPTER ONE

A is for Aspiration

Desire, longing, yearning.

Aspiration is, for many teachers, the root of how they began to put one foot in front of the other on the road to becoming a powerhouse teacher. With a little bit of help, anyone can learn to teach a sun salutation or give alignment suggestions, but certain teachers want to deeply effect change in their students and their communities. You may not have known it until you signed up for a teacher training or you may have dreamt it after your first class, but the aspiration to be a leader and share all that you have learned from your yoga practice started to expand somewhere along the way.

Unfortunately for teachers who share this vision and longing for greatness, there isn't a lot of support. We spend our teacher training programs learning the basics of teaching, not the art of being a great teacher or a powerful entrepreneur. Many teachers I have worked with over the years don't think of themselves as business people at all, which does not bode well for how they operate professionally. If you have ever felt the divide between your aspiration to be a successful teacher and the more practical side of your business, the following contemplation is for you.

Aspiration Exercise

Spend 5 minutes conjuring up the feelings of hope and ambition that helped you make the decision to embark on a yoga education.

Perhaps it struck you one day in Savasana as you listened to your teacher. Perhaps you had the realization when someone pointed out to you that you eat sleep and breathe yoga.

When did you feel called to walk this path?

What desire pulled you towards teaching that you couldn't ignore?

The powerful hunger that demanded to be fed was enough for you to arrange your time and make big changes to your life. Some part of you knew you *had* to teach yoga beyond all reason and doubt. Once you have sat with that energy for a few minutes, use it to look after something you have been putting off in your teaching life. It should be a simple task that you can look after in a matter of minutes.

Conjure up the power of aspiration to move something mundane forward every single day. Begin to connect the fact that to be a powerhouse teacher you must also embrace and care for the practical (and yes, sometimes boring) parts of your business.

CHAPTER TWO

B is for Business

It is always shocking to me how many teachers shy away from calling their work a "business." Many teachers can stand at the front of a room and perform the very complex task of guiding people through a physical, emotional and spiritual practice with total devotion, yet ironically don't put the same effort into promoting themselves so that *more* students can benefit from their expertise.

The idea of running a business might seem too big and official for you as an instructor, however, if you are getting paid to teach private or public classes it is time to face the music. It is understandable why you might not yet admit that you are a business owner and entrepreneur. It may be due to the fact that you love teaching so much, it is hard for you to take it seriously as a profession. Think of it this way, your "paid fun" is actually the best kind of business to have because you authentically enjoy it. That brand of passion touches people deeply and has the ability to carry you through the ups and downs of running said business.

If you decide to make teaching your full or part time career, adopting a business mentality is important. At some point you need to help your business thrive by spending more time building and nourishing it. As a teacher, part of the allure of this career is that your schedule deviates from the typical 9-5 and seems to lack the mile long "to-do" list. However, in order to run a successful business it is necessary to regularly check in and ensure you aren't dropping the ball due to your less traditional work hours.

One of the big traps I fell into early in my transition to a full time teacher, was buying into the notion that I only worked when I was teaching classes. My schedule had me up to teach a 6:30 am class after teaching until 9:30 or 10 pm the night before. Quickly I became exhausted, but my friends who worked during regular business hours could not understand why. Even if I taught fifteen classes each week, on paper it looked like half the number of working hours as my friends with conventional jobs. What I started to notice is that I spent another twenty hours per week on the *business* of my business without knowing, acknowledging and more importantly, without organizing my time well.

To be frank, I was very inefficient with my time. I would teach 3 classes in the same part of town, but didn't teach them on the same day (which would have saved two hours of driving every week). My work on my business was more like triage than prevention. I was flying by the seat of my pants for years and neglected project after project. It makes me cringe to think of how many people must have pigeon-holed me as a flaky yoga teacher (and probably for good reason).

When I got serious about making my teaching my livelihood, I knew I needed to become more professional. I outsourced the tasks I didn't want to do or wasn't qualified to do such as design work and invoicing. The most important routine I took on was setting aside time to work on my business with the same devotion I gave to my students in a class. The following exercise details the process I used to make my "business sessions" ultra-productive.

Exercise Your Business

Pick one day to work on the "business" of your business. You can do this weekly or monthly depending on your own needs, but know that this valuable time will shift your thinking and your output. On that day follow this process:

1) Begin by reviewing your big picture goals. It is important to write these down and put them somewhere you can see. Goals, especially big ones, need to be reinforced, and the best way to concretize the important things is to have a visual representation. If you want to include images and other objects that evoke the achievement of your goals, you'll find yourself with a potent "vision board."

2) Chart out the steps it may take to get you there. If your goal as a teacher is to open a yoga studio, such a daunting goal should be broken down into pieces. An example of some of the opening steps might include: speaking to a local studio owner about their experience, work with a commercial real estate agent to help you find a location, reach out to investors who can help you, formulate a business plan, take a course in opening a business, etc.

3) Give yourself deadlines for the bite sized steps towards your grand goals. Writing out your goals and breaking down the next steps is a major part of realizing them. Often you will feel great just for getting this far. It is important that you do not call it a day once you make it to this stage. This moment is the tricky part. I have worked with a lot of teachers that get to this point in their work, feel wonderful for having designed their next steps and deadlines and never do anything further.

4) Mark your deadlines on your calendar and stick to them.

5) Take time for your bookkeeping process. Pay your bills, invoice your clients and review your budget.

6) Finish off your session by dealing with any outstanding emails and phone calls.

CHAPTER THREE

C is for Connection

Now that you have started to gather energy from your original aspiration to become a yoga instructor and have begun to better monitor your business, it's time to explore how you connect.

Being a yoga teacher in the world right now is very exciting because there are so many ways of connecting with your student base. In the classroom the ways you engage with students are fairly straightforward. You might connect verbally, through physical adjustments, or by spending time meditating with your students during class. In the yoga space it is relatively easy to connect if you are a conscious and present person.

For students, the felt bond with you as their yoga teacher is very deep. Even if you don't exchange many words or know one another's background story, there is a powerful exchange that occurs during class. If you have not been in the role of student for some time you might forget how it feels to be in sync with the teacher as they guide you through your practice.

A successful yoga teacher weaves a special, magical quality into the fabric of their sessions because they know how to plug into the energy of each person in the room. Students will often remark that they feel as though their instructor is speaking only to them even if there are twenty other yogis in the space. Connection is more an art than a skill and one must be particularly attentive to ensure their teaching holds this weight on a regular basis.

Connection of course is not limited to the yoga mat. One of my favourite ways to stay connected to my students is through social media. Tools like <u>Facebook</u>, <u>Twitter</u> and <u>Instagram</u> allow you to share your insights about yoga, philosophy and the world with your students and your peers. However, I am always surprised to find that most teachers aren't utilizing these tools to the fullest, if at all.

Connect on Social Media

If you are a yoga teacher who avoids social media like the plague, let's begin with your argument. We all know that there is a lot of noise out there on web-based social platforms. We see celebrity scandals on Facebook, bitter feuds on Twitter and an overabundance of selfies on Instagram. The hype, the nonsense, and the lack of privacy and tact that have become the norm on social media platforms are enough to make anyone shy away from or shun these tools altogether.

From another perspective, if I told you there was a way to connect with your students daily through inspiring words, images and intriguing conversations wouldn't you be interested in investigating it?

As a yoga teacher, whether you are aware of it or not, you are a shining light in the noisy world of your students. They look to you and the space you provide for solace and a reprieve from their busy lives, which is why social media is one simple way for your students to remember how incredible you are and how fantastic they feel when they make room to practice.

The 10 Day Social Media Challenge

There is a teacher I mentor who once was a social media hater. I asked her to take the following challenge as an experiment:

1) Pick one social media outlet to use.

2) Each day, post or share something about yoga you find inspirational, interesting or better yet, relevant to your next yoga class or workshop (bonus points if you remind people to actually come to your class). Don't take more than 10 minutes each day to do it.

3) Respond to the comments if you have time.

One last thing: **Merely posting when and where you are teaching does not count.** Your posts must be authentically helpful or inspirational in order to be effective.

My lovely student begrudgingly agreed. After only one week of posting she called me to tell me that the responses she was getting were blowing her mind. People were engaging with her on Facebook suddenly. They were sharing her quotes and pictures with their friends. Students she hadn't seen in ages had re-emerged in her classes letting her know that her simple quote that day had been exactly what they needed to hear. One student said "I saw your quote and rearranged my day to be here because I just knew I needed to be in your class after that."

  If you aren't using social media to inspire and aid your students, there is no better time to start. I challenge every teacher I meet to do the social media challenge because otherwise you may never know how many people you can reach with an insight that seems second nature to you. Luckily, with the ease of connecting on social platforms, you will probably hear back from many of the people you touch. At worst, you might start a beautiful conversation, at best you might find an untapped source for filling your classes and being more successful.

CHAPTER FOUR

D is for Direction

I define being a successful yoga teacher as bringing together masterful instruction, a deep understanding of yoga and a soulful love of building a sustainable business. As you work through the contemplations and experiments in this book, you will notice that there are many small things you can work on without a large commitment of time and resources. These small projects have been paired with mighty insights to help you realize your full power and purpose.

As a yoga teacher, you may not give much value to having a precise direction for your business. In fact, you may be so busy tending to the smaller details of your weekly schedule, that you haven't thought to chart your way towards a particular goal. You may indeed enjoy the simplicity of living life from day to day and crafting your time almost any way you want. That is a perk of being a yoga teacher after all.

Not a morning person? You can set your schedule to start later in the day.

Love to teach get up early and practice? You can book yourself up for daytime classes exclusively and be in bed at 9pm.

Many teachers don't map out a clear direction for their business because they tend to be a more laid back with a "go with the flow" attitude than the average business owner. As healthy as that can be in certain situations, it can also work against you if you aren't consciously invested in one direction over another. For instance, if you know you eventually want to open a studio, the smaller choices in your career need to be moving you in that direction.

Does it make sense to travel 7 months a year teaching if your goal is to set up shop in the town you live in? Or should you invest your time in learning about admin and studio management and work on building relationships within your community?

Knowing the general direction in which you would like to move is a major factor in success. And learning how to say "no" to things that don't move you in your desired direction is just as important as saying "yes" to the things that do.

Written Direction Exercise

In order to plot your course and next steps as a teacher, work through the following exercise regularly. Set up a monthly date with yourself in your calendar so you can stay flexible and reflect on your direction.

1) When you dream about where you want your work as a teacher to go, what does it look like? Think big goals and dreams.

2) What choices are you making that result in progress in that direction? Pat yourself on the back here. Celebrate the little things as well as the big!

3) Where are you leaking energy on projects that don't support your direction? Name all the parts of your work that make you groan or exhaust you.

4) How can you plug the energy leaks on those projects? Think creatively on how you can avoid the "groaners" from now on.

CHAPTER FIVE

E is for Empowered Evaluation

Once you have set your sights on your goal and begin to move forward in that direction, it is important to set yourself up with some ground rules to facilitate the follow through. Yoga attracts people who are creatively gifted and led by their hearts to champion its wisdom into the future. Sadly, in moments where the heart leaps to say "yes" to a new opportunity, it often overrides the rational mind.

The rational mind lends a great deal to decision making. It can act as the dispassionate, more objective, voice of reason--weighing pros and cons, looking at the facts and taking into account known history around the choice at hand. And yet somewhere along the way in the yoga world, we have developed a major stigma against the rational mind. The division between "using your head" and "following your heart" is very real for many yoga instructors.

My life certainly didn't follow the traditional path of my contemporaries. I spent most of my childhood summers in theatre camps, more interested in singing and acting than sports. A month before I was supposed to ship off to university, I discovered I was only going because society said I was *supposed* to, and after a brief examination of my personal values and goals at the time, I decided instead to attend a one year intensive program for music recording and engineering.

A series of twists and turns during my career led me to take a yoga teacher training and, after some years, I decided to jump from the music business into teaching full time. While I built my teaching business, I completed a four-year course in acupuncture and Chinese medicine. After several years of life running a successful part time clinic and a very busy teaching business, I gave up everything and moved to the U.S. to begin a new chapter with my partner.

Reading this might make one think:

(a) She is an irrational, hot mess who couldn't stick to one thing or got bored after things became routine.
or:
 (b) She is a free spirit who followed her heart and decided not to live her life according to someone else's rules.

"Rational" people usually agree with the first statement. "Follow Your Heart" people tend to believe the second.

The truth of course is a mix of both. There have certainly been times where my rational mind has kept me from taking a scary leap into the unknown only to regret it later. Similarly, I have "followed my heart" off of several cliffs.

What I gained from all the mistakes and troubles I have experienced so far ,however, is the insight that the head and heart *must* operate together more often than not to avoid disaster.

How does this relate to the business of teaching?

When I ask teachers what their main obstacle is along the path towards success, the most common answer by far is **lack of time**.

"There aren't enough hours in the day!"

"My goals are taking up more time than I have."

"I can't seem to fit it all in."

Digging a little deeper, it is quickly revealed that most (though not all) of the busy-ness is self-inflicted. The heart leaps at an opportunity and most yoga teachers make decisions on the momentary inspiration. While it feels good in the moment, they simultaneously eschew the supposed oppression of the rational mind's doubt and judgment. Teachers who make rationality the enemy and only do what their hearts cry out for, will inevitably drop the ball, let people down and screw up.

Why does this happen?

If you make your head the enemy of the heart you will tend to make promises based on one singular factor, a happy moment. It is so easy to project a good feeling into the future without working through all details, including the time or energy it will take to execute the process.

If you have ever found yourself in this situation, I implore you to reconsider a ceasefire with your rational mind. Some people will tell you that if you spend too much time examining a decision your heart is yearning to make, you are opening the door to fear and self-doubt. It's easy to confuse the process of over thinking something and stirring up your worst nightmares with rational thought. Let's be very clear here: you can tell when your thought process is wracked with fear and doubt rather than rational thinking by its emotional weight. The former is heavy, while the latter should be a no-drama process that takes into account both what your wild heart wants and what is practical for you to give.

Empowered Evaluation

The next time someone asks you to do anything business related, whether the request is to teach at a new studio or drive for an hour to lead a meditation session, implement the Empowered Evaluation process.

1) Press Pause. If you tend to say yes to every opportunity that makes your heart leap, instead respond with "Let me get back to you on that."

2) Let the decision rest for at least 24 hours and then ask yourself, Is this opportunity:

- Something I want to do because it is fun, exciting etc.?
- Supporting a friend or cause I believe in?
- Aligned with my direction and big goals?
- Something I have the time/energy for?

If you can't honestly answer, "yes" (with both heart and rational mind in agreement) to at least two of these questions, politely decline and save that precious time and energy.

Practice saying "Let me get back to you" on everything you are asked for a full week. Notice the times you might normally over-commit and later regret after thinking through the obligations it will place on you. You don't need to do this exercise forever (unless you find it helpful), do it for as long as it takes until you can use both rational thinking and conscious attention to make better directional decisions.

CHAPTER SIX

F is for Failure

Hold the phone. FAILURE?!

That's right. Learning how to fail is an important part of being a business owner and a teacher. The willingness to take a risk, try new things and be flexible enough to change directions is actually a spiritual practice for yoga teachers. Even those of us who have mastered the skill to use both head and heart as trusted advisors in all decisions, know that some ventures simply won't work out.

The risk of taking on a new class at an awkward time slot means you have to roll the dice on something that could be a total flop. Getting out of your comfort zone to teach a specialized workshop or lead a weekend retreat requires a lot of work, planning and showing off your beloved new offering. There is a chance, maybe a big one, that your next offering will fail.

The problem isn't failure. That is bound to happen now and then. The problem is how you deal with it. The most common conclusion of an instructor whose class has flopped is "my community doesn't love me, I am a terrible teacher and no one values what I have to offer." A more helpful response should be, "Well that experiment didn't work, I wonder if I promoted this well, picked a good time slot or offered something people really want."

In the <u>Yoga Teacher Survival Course</u>, I interviewed my friend and studio owner Katie McClelland. She said that in her early days, she taught over 1000 classes with less than 5 people in them. Now she owns three successful studios in my hometown and has helped build a thriving yoga community. Imagine what would have happened if she had closed up shop after a few weeks of slow classes instead of learning how to build her business.

I know the failure issue is a deep one for many yoga teachers. You put your heart and soul into your classes and offerings and if they don't succeed the way you had hoped, it is difficult not to take it personally. The exercise that follows is adapted from my e-book on teaching private yoga. It will help you lick your wounds and get back in the game when things fail.

Failure Analysis Exercise

Something about your teaching isn't working. Your class numbers are dwindling, your workshop doesn't have people signed up or you aren't getting enough classes to fill your schedule.

1) Have an honest, no-drama evaluation of the situation with yourself. Are you consistently bringing your best teaching self to your classes? Are you present with your students, offering them as much of your knowledge as possible? What external factors are playing in to this failure? Did your endeavor lack proper promotion or administration?

2) Focus on the positive lessons to be learned. Once you figure out the main issues, chart out what you will you do differently the next time to get a different outcome. Think of each failure as an experiment and try changing some of the factors for the next round until you find a new formula with a better result.

Things to Remember:

Yoga is for everyone, but your class might not be. If you find you are truly mismatched with a group of students or an event, find a better fit. Move on as quickly and cleanly as possible.

If this were easy everyone would do it. Making a living as a teacher takes time, effort and the ability to stay strong even during slow periods and transitions. If you allow yourself to be shaken with every tough moment it will be hard to move forward with confidence. When failure happens, take time to remember your big picture goals and keep your focus there.

CHAPTER SEVEN

G is for Gratitude

*"At times our own light goes out and is rekindled
by the spark from another person. Each of us
has cause to think with deep gratitude of those
who have lighted the flame within us."*
~Albert Schweitzer

The above quote reminds me of the many teachers who have rekindled my own flame along the yogic path. The magic and mystery of teaching is that you come together with students to move them through a practice that works in unseen ways on their psyches. You don't know if they are at a class after a long hard day, trying to improve their health or if they are hungry for a life with more depth. You may never know what insights they are having or what they might be battling with.

The space you hold and the words you speak affect your students. But how does your personal felt sense of gratitude play in and how does it make you successful?

One of the keys of being a successful yoga teacher is directly influenced by the attitude you bring to your classes. Since the teacher is responsible for crafting the space in which the student practices, nothing makes a class fall flat like an instructor who isn't totally present. If you have started to take your teaching for granted and you no longer connect with what a privilege it is to teach, there will be a sharp palpable edge to your classes.

I attended a class recently where the teacher, let's call her Jen, led us through a moderately challenging practice, using a very contrived yoga teacher voice. We all know it is important to be loud, clear and not rush while teaching a class, but her voice was one of those fake "I am the yoooooga teacher" ones that drives me up the wall. To make things worse, Jen made unnecessary and downright cynical comments about how difficult each posture was at least once every 5 minutes. She didn't leave her mat more than twice, gave no adjustments and barely seemed to look at any of the 30+ people in the room.

Her attitude came off as casual and disinterested and instead of guiding me, she was distracting me. I found myself ripping my attention off my breath and out of the pose and on to her negative commentary about how "rough" the class was and how much we probably all hated her.

I know a burned out teacher when I see one and Jen was surely that.

Teach for long enough and you will inevitably go through times when your well is dry. It can be tempting to go on autopilot when energy is low or while dealing with personal upheaval. This has happened to me more times than I can count in my career. The solution isn't always easy, but it starts with **cultivating more gratitude.**

Remember, your students didn't show up to hear how bad your day was or to make you feel better. They came to your class to learn from you and be guided. Never disrespect that level of trust by going in with a negative or entitled attitude.

Gratitude Exercise

Without being inauthentic about your momentary reality, use these simple techniques to remind you daily to treasure the life you have been afforded.

1) Before you start teaching, spend 5 minutes recalling a time that a yoga class lifted you out of a tough day. Conjure up the feeling of gratitude towards the practice and let it infuse your own class.

2) Keep a gratitude journal. Name at least 5 things you are grateful for each day.

3) A common yoga favourite is to invite your entire class to dedicate their practice to someone or something they feel deep gratitude towards. Stay attentive while you teach in honour of that intention.

Students will always find it more inspiring to be around a teacher who is grateful. Since being a successful teacher hinges on people wanting to work with you and take your classes, it makes sense that you take on a gratitude practice as part of your own development.

CHAPTER EIGHT

H is for Harmony

When I went to school for Chinese Medicine one of my instructors destroyed my favourite yoga buzz word at the time: balance. He pointed out that the obsession with the modern concept of balance (considered the crowning achievement of all health-conscious people) was actually the ultimate stagnation.

The very foundation of life in the body depends not on balance but homeostasis which is a constant fluctuation that internally stabilizes and regulates important processes of the body. ***To be balanced he said, meant that these tiny movements had ceased and life had ended.***

In another domain, you have no doubt heard the term "work/life balance" that many students strive for and come to yoga help to find. I have seen the obsession with this misinterpreted, so-called "balance" get pretty twisted. From students that work a stressful job 10+ hours a day and think that a one hour yoga class should erase the negative effects of that lifestyle, to people who eat a mound of processed foods and sugars and believe they can "balance" it out with a salad... tomorrow.

The struggle and obsession with "balance" is often dis-empowering and has been dangled in front of us for too long.

Instead of seeking balance, I encourage you to find harmony. This concept allows for the natural cycles of life to be as they are while introducing a healthier flux and a more worthy pursuit. The quest for harmony gives permission to the seeker to acknowledge that during certain phases you may need to work longer hours in order to get your career on track. It allows for more sleep and rest when you are feeling under the weather. Building a harmonious life places the responsibility to make better choices, more often, on the individual.

Balance feels like struggling to reach a certain point then holding your breath and hoping nothing changes.

Harmony takes into consideration the ups and downs of life and what is needed moment to moment in order to bring vibrancy.

Harmony Contemplation

Spend time examining the difference between balance and harmony for yourself.

Are you chasing after a perfectly balanced life, or a more harmonious one when it comes to success?

Is there a way in your teaching you can promote more harmony and less stagnation for your students?

Journal this for yourself or discuss your insights in the Facebook group: Being a Successful Yoga Teacher

CHAPTER NINE

I is for Ideal Client

One familiar refrain I give over and over again to yoga teachers is, "yoga is for everyone, but your class might not be." This small but mighty insight has helped many of the teachers I work with begin to recognize that they don't need to waste time and energy trying to be a one-size-fits-all instructor. More importantly, it has freed up the space for these teachers to ask themselves "Who is my Ideal Client or Student?".

For over a decade, the core of my teaching business has been small group or one-on-one private classes. Yet many teachers I work with find the arena of private classes to be mysterious and untouchable. What makes this problematic is the fact that leading private classes is one of the only ways to make teaching yoga a sustainable career choice. It is my strongly held belief that if you are teaching more than 15 classes a week you are walking a path that will lead to burnout.

The 3 Keys to Finding and Keeping Your Ideal Students

1) Clarity

The first key to finding and keeping your ideal students is to know who they are. I spend one full class on this in the Yoga Teacher Survival Course because it is shocking how many teachers have a hard time with getting clear on who they want to help and how.

To understand who your Ideal Clients are, ask yourself:

What do I enjoy teaching most? (Flow, Yin, Restorative, Yoga for Athletes, Yoga Therapy)

What types of people are attracted to this form of yoga?

Dream up one or two personas that best describe the people you want to work with in a private setting. When I created Aquin Yoga, I spent several days working on the persona of my readers and Ideal Clients. To help get you started, answer the following questions:

What is your Ideal Client's profession?
What do they do for fun?
What do they value in life?
What are they passionate about?
Why are they interested in Yoga?
What do they want to learn?
What qualities are they looking for in an instructor?

Spend time gaining clarity on who you most want to work with and it will inform everything about how you approach those people and what you do together.

2) Connection

Now that you are clear on who your Ideal Clients are, the second key is to connect with them. While there are many ways to do this effectively, blogging is a phenomenal vehicle of connection with your students. When I first began, I hated the idea of blogging and had to be lovingly strong-armed into it by my co-founder Steve Haase. Marketing master that he is, he pointed out that I had already built loyalty from my ideal students because of the content I shared while teaching, but the only way those people had found me was by stumbling into my class one day. Without an online voice, I was missing the chance to connect with Ideal Clients all over the world.

Sharing your ideas, tips and love for yoga through writing and video allows your students to see who you are and what gets you fired up. If those people love what you do and appreciate what you are offering, they will stay connected and engaged. People who are connected and engaged are more likely to take the next step and become a lifelong student who will also share your work with their friends and family.

You don't need a fancy website with all the bells and whistles; something simple, like a blog that allows for the exchange of thoughts between you and your ideal students, is enough to get you started.

3) Consistency

Once you are clear and connected to your ideal students, the final key comes into play. Being a consistent teacher doesn't sound sexy, but I can assure you it is hands down **the most important factor in keeping ongoing classes with your ideal students**.

Nothing annoys me more than when a teacher jumps erratically between styles of yoga in order to "shake things up" when truthfully, they just trying to keep things interesting for themselves at the expense of their students. As instructors, we should be refining our teaching skills and striving towards innovation, but there is no need to be all over the place for no reason.

My background in yoga is rooted in the Ashtanga Vinyasa world so I appreciate the power of structure and routine through repetition of the same postures. However, I am constantly trying to find creative yet logical transitions and progressions in and out of a handful of postures I consider fundamental. After years of teaching, I have learned that it takes skill and guts to walk in to a room with the only lesson plan being working with who shows up to class and what shows up in my brain that day. In order to stay fresh and have the class feel consistent try:

1) Having a framework, even a loose and flexible one, for your time with your students.

2) Ending the class the same way each time no matter what the contents of the class (I always end with a 10 minute savasana).

3) Picking an apex pose to work on each week until it is a familiar to the student and integrated into the practice.

4) Returning to a core theme or idea throughout the class.

These three keys to finding and keeping your ideal students are not a magic formula, but if you work with them they will help to improve your business. Don't overlook the importance of getting clear on who you really want to be working with. This will dictate all the decisions big and small on how you operate your business and the way you teach.

CHAPTER TEN

J is for Join

We all know that yoga means to yoke or unite. And yet sadly for many teachers, the yoga world isn't always as inviting as one would hope. When I began teaching, I was shocked at how many teachers were engaging in non-yogic behaviour. Jealousy and petty misunderstandings so frequently infected studios I attended that I quickly became disillusioned. I didn't see the teamwork and yoking my own instructors had promoted during my training. I saw instead shrewd, manipulative tactics and positioning that I naively believed only existed in the corporate world.

This is a dirty little secret existent in so many pockets of the yoga industry.

In fact, it has become a passionate mission of mine to unite teachers in a way that is warm and professional so everyone can thrive and develop without looking over their shoulders afraid someone is going to undercut or take away business.

A Race to the Bottom

Fear and jealousy are the main reasons that so many studios are on a race to the bottom in terms of their pricing for classes. Sadly, popular thinking and lack of real business knowledge has led a major percentage of studio owners and freelance teachers to engage in a practice of undercutting one another.

Typically when a new studio opens even remotely near another, it kick starts a cycle of fear and jealousy. The new studio owner, afraid of being the new kid on the block offers a drastic promotion like a month of free yoga. Most often the owner has no financial backing of any kind and has never run a business before. They simply love yoga and have a beautiful dream.

While they are offering this promotion they ask their new teachers to "be a team" and take no payment or a very meager sum to help build up the studio. Some teachers do this willingly, not realizing that this is actually a bigger issue.

Think about it. If you went to work at a retail store or restaurant that was just opening and they asked you to work without being paid for the first month until things got busier, you wouldn't do it. In fact if anyone asked you to do such a thing, the labour laws of your country would have something to say. Some yoga studios however do not pay their teachers during this time and justify it as a promotional period. Owners may go so far as to spin this as a way for new teachers to get exposure, which sounds better than what it really is: unpaid labour.

Meanwhile, the more established studios start to panic. There is a shiny new studio in town with a fresh energetic owner who hasn't been run down from years of having to deal with interpersonal issues with the staff and the demands of students.

What if the new space is nicer?

What if their teachers are better?
What if everyone likes them more?

Full of fear and jealousy, the more experienced owner offers a loyalty discount and undercuts the drop in rate of the new studio by a few bucks. Naturally the new studio begins to counter by cutting their prices and not paying teachers their promised salary as they struggle to keep the lights on.

Meanwhile, the established studio starts to cut corners to save money. They begin to only hire teachers fresh out of training because they can hire them for next to nothing. They also stop holding workshops with master teachers because they cost more (even though the studio is known for hosting interesting and innovative teachers). When the numbers start to drop they blame it on the new studio without considering the possibility that their clients are leaving because they feel the quality of the studio declining.

Fear and jealousy are so strong that these two

owners, both feeling much the same thing, can never reach out to one another for support.

Potential

You might have been a player in some variation of this story since you began teaching. I don't need to tell you how toxic and degrading it feels. And yet at some point before you witnessed a version of this tale, there was a sense that running your own business as a teacher or studio owner had the potential to be very fulfilling.

The lack of camaraderie and trust between teachers in many communities leaves much to be desired, which is why you need teammates to get you motivated. In truth, there is no reason you cannot create a healthy group of instructors to nourish your work and your business. If you aren't sure how, start with this simple challenge.

Join Exercise: The "Show Some Love" Challenge

Joining together with other teachers is the best way to support and inspire each other as you work towards your big goals. Ask any successful person you know and they will tell you (if they are humble enough) that they couldn't have made it without the enormous support and generosity of others. In the spirit of unity that *is* the heart of yoga, team up with another teacher to build success together. Here's one way:

1) Pick a yoga teacher that you admire.

2) Share their poster (or Facebook event, workshop info, etc.) on social media or in an email to your student base with a personal testimonial as to how much you love their work.

3) Let the teacher know you did it and suggest an in-person meeting or phone call to talk about your mutual goals and how you might support one another's big goals.

Don't think of this as some networking technique (which can come across as cold and self-serving) because you aren't asking for anything in return. You are simply giving support and making room for a new potential. As such, make sure you feel authentically connected to the other instructor and start to build a relationship based on mutual respect, creative inspiration and mad yoga love.

CHAPTER ELEVEN

K is for Karma

My actions are my only true belongings. I cannot escape the consequences of my actions. My actions are the ground upon which I stand.
~Thích Nhất Hạnh

Karma, or the sum of one's actions, is something you have no doubt learned about as a student and teacher of yoga. But have you ever thought about how it pertains to your business?

When I finished my first 250-hour teacher training I was blown away by the amount of pettiness and greed corrupting the yoga world. Some of the teachers I adored disappointed me by trashing their peers or sleeping with their students. The story of fear and jealousy I described in the last chapter played out many times right before my eyes as I discovered studios I used to love and dreamed of teaching at were withholding paychecks or forcing teachers to teach for free for months as a "probation" period.

In those first few years, I witnessed a lot of bad karma being accumulated and distributed. Because of it, I got lost in a cloud of cynicism that caused me to be very protective of my own classes and careful about who I trusted.

The sad truth hidden in many corners of the yoga world is that most schools, studios and teachers don't practice what they preach.

It is rare to see one teacher share helpful tools with another, let alone rave about another instructor's class or share someone else's work with their students. Sadly this creates isolation and an "every man for himself" mentality that eats away at would-be healthy yoga communities.

If you don't think this negative collective karma is affecting you, let me ask you this: **Did you perform the "Show Love" challenge yet?**

If you did, then great!
If not, why did you feel resistance to support another teacher?

Moving forward and burning up that karma is one of the most important things you can do to be truly successful. Here are some points to contemplate to get you started.

Abundance is not finite
Do you deeply believe that there is only so much success to go around? If so, just remember yoga has reached millions of people, but there are so many more who haven't found the right style, teacher or path yet. Since you can't possibly be everything to everyone, embrace and cheer on other instructors as they serve their own ideal students and clients.

There is no competition
Even if you live in a huge yoga market, the only way you can be in competition with anyone is to engage in it. Only you can offer your special brand of yoga in just the way you do, so allow your teaching to be a practice for you and your

students, not a sporting event between you and the studio down the road. The most successful studio I have worked with makes it a point to welcome new studios in the area when they open. The owner often goes to the open house of a new studio with flowers and congratulations. They also barter for free classes for the teachers between studios so everyone can get to know and respect one another.

Practice what you preach
What is the theme of your teaching? Is it unity, growth, self-awareness, health, strength, devotion, gratitude? Whatever your main message, keep your eye on the prize in all instances. Run your business as an example of your main theme with no compromise. Undercutting another teacher to get a new class, gossiping, being insincere or dishonest is never worth the price you will pay in the end.

Broken trust is the disease of the yoga world and something we all need to help deal with both practically and karmically
The only way to burn up this negative karma is to

create new patterns and habits and the only one to do it is you. Take responsibility for things you have done in the past that were not in alignment with your highest principles. While no one can change the past, we can often repair the damage in some way and commit to a new way of operating.

CHAPTER TWELVE

L is for Longevity

Have you ever considered your longevity as a yoga teacher?

Success in any profession depends on being able to sustain a high level of quality output for an extended period of time. If you can't keep up and deliver the goods, any "success" you achieve will be short lived and likely followed by a burnout period.

I have seen a multitude of teachers crank out fifteen or more classes a week for years on end. Some burn out catastrophically and quit teaching forever. More commonly, I observe stress and overflowing schedules subtly eat away at healthy people. These teachers seem to get sick every other month, lose their sparkle and start subbing out more classes than they teach.

My own insight on longevity struck me in the winter of 2013. I was teaching 11-12 classes and running my part time acupuncture clinic every week when I caught a low grade cold that lasted almost a month. It wasn't bad enough for me to to miss work so I just plowed through. By February I noticed some stiffness in one knee that began spreading to other joints all over my body.

Fast forward to a few months later when I was diagnosed with rheumatoid arthritis, an autoimmune disease that has no known cure. Not only did this wreak havoc on my life emotionally and physically, it caused me to take stock of my own longevity as a teacher.

We can break longevity down in a few different ways. One deals with the physical realm. While you can't control every aspect of your health (my circumstance is proof of that), you do control much of what goes into fueling your vehicle. Ensuring a healthy diet, ample sleep, as well as a sustainable yoga and fitness practice all nourish your physical well-being.
You also need emotional health and spiritual longevity to keep the party going. Taking at least

a full day off each week, going on regular retreats or vacations, meditating and making time for people who love, support and inspire you, all beautify your internal landscape.

The Yin and Yang of Self Care

When you hear the phrase "self-care" do you think about warm baths or buying yourself flowers? If you enjoy those things then that might be one aspect of your self care routine, but as anyone who works alongside other human beings knows, self-care means so much more.

One dimension of self-care is the more traditional version (the warm baths and flowers route). This is considered the Yin form as it is nurturing and enveloping. Yin self-care is what the person who loves you most in the world does for you when you are having a rough day or feeling sick, encircling you with warm fuzzies.

Another aspect of self-care is the Yang dimension. It's the type of care that a coach or mentor might deliver. It is positivity that pushes you forward and doesn't let you hold back your potential. Yang self-care doesn't let you eat cookie dough on the sofa while you watch your favourite childhood movie for the millionth time, it gets you off your butt and out to the gym or to yoga.

One is not better than the other, they are just different aspects of the same thing. Here are some examples:

Yin Self Care

Going to bed early so you can get a full 7-8 hrs of sleep.

Taking a sanity break, free from phone calls and email.

Spending time with loved ones enjoying a long meal.

Reading a novel.

Yang Self Care

Getting up early in the morning to do a physical practice.

Spending a day pushing through outstanding

work so you can relax on the weekend.
Spending time with loved ones working out, or
doing some healthy activity.
Learning a new skill or hobby.

Yin is nurturing and recharging. Yang is inspiring
and developmental. And both are extremely
important to our health and well-being.

  As human beings, we have to be aware that we
have the tendency to favour one type over the
other. Those who favour Yin self-care tend to
judge Yang forms as being too aggressive or
busy and therefore not self-care at all. Those
who lean more towards Yang self-care may view
Yin forms as being lazy and indulgent. While
both are true when not tempered by the other,
developing your self-awareness will help you to
assess what you need at different times.

If you have worked a fifty hour week and slept no
more than 6 hours a night, some Yin self-care
might be in order. If things have been light in
your schedule but you still feel underlying stress
or the need for something more, a dose of Yang

is the fire you need. The inner dimensions of life feed the outer and vice versa, so adding a splash of self-care will do wonders for you. As a teacher you are your business, so that which nourishes you will filter through and make you a more available and awesome yoga instructor.

Self Care for Longevity Guidelines

There is no hard and fast rule to determine what your self-care regime might include, but I will offer a few simple guidelines that apply to both Yin and Yang self-care.

1) If it doesn't fuel you or nourish you, it isn't self-care.

2) Self-care means you do it for yourself. While we sometimes need to ask for help in our lives, self-care should be empowering and something you can do for yourself with as little reliance elsewhere as possible (except of course for things like body work or health treatments where you put yourself in someone's care for a time).

3) Self-care is something you look forward to. If you don't enjoy it or otherwise get a deep benefit, it won't fuel or nourish you.

4) Self-care results in health and vitality. Self-care does not mean going out and eating a 3-

layer cake or getting bombed. Never use self-care to justify bad habits or behaviour that hurts you or anyone else.

5) Self-care is necessary to your well-being. Take it seriously.

Did you catch that last one? **Self-care is necessary to your well-being. Take it seriously.**

This is your life, and if you are a responsible, awake individual (or at the very least, want to become one) self-care is part of your work to make sure you are firing on all cylinders.

CHAPTER THIRTEEN

M is for Marketing

In all the coaching and training I have done with yoga instructors, nothing feels like pulling teeth more than work around marketing and self-promotion. Somehow in this profession, people who can hold the attention of a room and speak confidently while giving adjustments seem to shrink at the prospect of mentioning their next workshop at the end of a class. If you despise marketing and eschew self-promotion, I beg you not to skip this section or its exercise.

Marketing is such a big and important topic that I couldn't possibly cover it all in one chapter. I will, however, share a powerful idea that has helped the teachers I work with in the past when they were kicking and screaming against marketing and self-promotion.

You are a yoga teacher. You have seen beyond cultural norms and have found a world that allows you to explore life outside of the bounds of consumerism. You know that no one wants posters on their car, spam in their email or a phone call during dinner from someone trying to sell something. These outdated practices not only cost more than they are worth, but they enrage the people you are trying to reach.

Think of all the times an advertisement or cheap marketing tactic has annoyed you so much that you vowed never to use the product again!

On the other hand, *you are a yoga teacher who wants to be successful*, not only in your teaching but also financially. A great teacher isn't doing anyone any favours by keeping all of their work to themselves. You could be the best teacher on the planet but you can't help anyone if you don't have students.

In order to develop a thriving student base, you need to tell people how to find you. You must offer things your "Ideal Client" is interested in so that you can nurture their learning. All of that takes time and resources, so you must also be appropriately compensated.

Marketing and self-promotion can be as simple as sharing with your students what your next class is and why it will be beneficial, fun or educational. One of the teachers I coach recently proved that this simple technique works by mentioning her upcoming retreat at the end of every class. This gifted woman had almost given up on her offering when we started working together. She had decided a month before the retreat that she wouldn't have enough people to run it and that her students were probably sick of seeing the posters all over the studio or in the newsletter.

I convinced her to write a few of the key benefits the retreat would deliver and practice talking about it from a student-centered perspective. After just a week of doing this in every class, her retreat filled up and blew her expectations out of the water!

Inbound Marketing

What I find so interesting is that most yoga teachers are already masters at one of the most modern and amazing marketing practices I have found to date. The marketing technique is called Inbound Marketing. The basic premise is that rather than interrupting someone's day with an irrelevant ad (the old way of doing things), you build a relationship with your potential clients based on their level of interest and by sharing authentically useful things with them.

Teaching yoga offers a very special opportunity to forge genuine connections and share your message with a captive audience in each and every class. The position of the student is a vulnerable one. Learning something new isn't easy and your students have consciously made the decision to show up in your world and put themselves in your hands. What's more, each time you adjust your students both physically and verbally, you let them know they are seen and cared for.

Powerful, effective marketing makes the audience feel seen and understood. They feel truly engaged and if it is exceptional, they feel like someone has their own best interests in mind. The most effective yoga teachers I know make me feel this way when I am in their class, and when I find out they are offering a workshop or retreat I jump at the opportunity to spend more time with them. The trust you build with your students will result in this same feeling because there's a whole world of people who already love yoga and are looking for the unique experience you bring to their lives.

Simple Non-Cheesy, Non-Sleazy Marketing

The next time you feel awkward about mentioning an upcoming class or workshop, run through these points. Practice speaking about your offerings until you feel confident.

1) What and When: "Before you leave class, I wanted to mention that I am teaching a Yoga for Runners Workshop here next Saturday at 2pm."

2) Why should they go: "This is one of my most popular workshops and it will be focused on the essential stretches and strengthening runners need to be their best. We will also have time to go over your personal issues in your running followed by a beautiful integrative Savasana."

3) Why should they sign up right now: "There are only 10 spots left," "The early bird discount ends tomorrow," "Space is limited," "It is a lot of fun so it sells out quickly."

Personal touch: "It is my favourite workshop to teach so I hope you can join me." "If you have any questions please let me know."

CHAPTER FOURTEEN

N is for Nurture

Yoga teachers are generally excellent nurturers, which is an important feature of being a good marketer. Even if you aren't the warm fuzzy "Earth Mama" type, you either have a natural gift, or have done the work to learn the skill that allows you to assist others to grow. Whatever your teaching style, you know that the key to staying in business depends on a healthy client base of people who are willing to pay you to teach them. Students pay you because you have knowledge that they can benefit from.

While you pat yourself on the back for being so darn wonderful, you might wonder why, if you are already an expert at nurturing people and their yoga practice, you need this lesson in the first place. One of the keys to being a successful yoga teacher is learning how to nurture your students in a way that helps them make it to class more often and enrich their practice.

The Typical Model

In the business world, companies spend a lot of time tracking the ways strangers turn into customers. It costs time, money and manpower to make this happen and it is important for studio owners and private teachers to to examine this channel more closely. The common strategy (and one I am not a fan of) is to offer new student specials that studios use to get people in the door.

This tactic is now the norm in most major centres because almost every studio does it. However, no studio could possibly survive if all its members only paid thirty dollars per month. The aim of such a drastic promotion is that using this low cost incentive will ideally get new people in the door where they will proceed to fall in love with the studio, the teachers, and the community.

For certain studios with a big budget and who work in an unsaturated market, this method has helped build their business, but for independent teachers I urge you not to reduce your rates. The more teachers continue to do this, the more dangerous it becomes to work as a professional in this industry. It is time for instructors to stop trying to outdo one another in a race to the bottom of the pricing barrel.

How to Nurture Sustainably

If you aren't going to compete with the bargain basement rates other teachers are hurting their businesses over, what should you do to keep your bank account happy?

The smart move for both studios and independent teachers is to spend time nurturing pre-existing students.

I mentioned that a savvy pro can tell you the average cost of acquiring a new client, but in most cases, the cost of keeping an existing client is far less than finding a new one. My own teaching practice was built on referrals, as were those of most of the other successful teachers I know. When you tailor your classes or studio to your ideal clients, you will attract students who become loyal fans. Your new loyal fans will be eager to bring their friends who become fans as well. This process depends on teaching consistent classes and truly valuing the people who are regular students.

Most studios and teachers focus a lot of time and effort on acquiring new students and, as such, neglect the consistent and loyal people. I remember running into a student a few years ago who had once been a regular client of a studio I taught at. This one person had personally brought well over twenty friends (many of whom became monthly members) over the years to the studio. I was thrilled to see her and interested to know why she had been absent from her mat for so long.

She told me that while she loved the teachers at the studio, she was fed up that there seemed to be consistent revolving door "new student" incentives that flooded her favourite classes for months at a time. She said she was tired of fighting for a spot in the room with people who were paying on average less than five dollars a class and didn't respect the culture and etiquette of the studio. More than that, she felt that she wasn't able to progress in her own practice because the instructor's attention was on assisting the newer students.

It made sense to me why she felt slighted. She had given so much of her time, effort and hard-earned money over the years and expected that the studio would uphold its end of the commitment and provide her with consistent, high quality classes in a well-managed space. She had lost faith in the mission of the studio and felt they only cared to pack more people into classes to make more money and no longer cared about her safety and progress.

As with any relationship, if you only pay attention and go out of your way to make the other person happy at the beginning they probably won't stick around once they feel neglected.

Exercises in Nurturing

The good news for yoga teachers is that you probably already deeply care for the people who come to your classes regularly and already give them all you have in the classroom. Nurturing your current clients off the mat simply means you give them added fuel now and then. You don't need to do anything flashy or invest a fortune into nurturing your students. Here are some very simple things you can do:

- Send out an inspirational email to your students.

- Spend a few minutes before or after class speaking with them (stay professional but be informal).

- Check in via email if you know they have been ill or dealing with personal issues (again, keep it pro).

- Send a birthday message to your students.

- Share an amusing or educational yoga-related video or article periodically.

- If you offer new client incentives, offer a loyalty incentive for your pre-existing clients.

- If your clients refer you elsewhere, thank them with a handwritten card or small token of appreciation such as a small bottle of savasana oil, homemade bath salts or beeswax candles.

Connecting with your students isn't just good for your business, it feeds their soul to hear from someone they admire, and it will feed yours to be in touch with your wonderful students and nurture them both on and off the mat.

CHAPTER FIFTEEN

O is for Organization

A major difficulty for many yoga instructors is organization (or lack thereof). Although often overlooked, being disorganized is the most underrated blockage towards true success.

Here is a quick test to see how organized you really are. Answer honestly.

1) On a daily basis do you misplace your: keys, wallet, phone?

2) When you go shopping, do you get home and realize you have forgotten something on your list?

3) Do you have a lot of clutter or mystery boxes in your home?

4) Does your "to do" list fill you with anxiety?

5) Do you forget appointments or show up late to

classes or to teach?

If you answered yes to even one of these questions, chances are that it's time for a pattern break.

As a yoga teacher, you may easily put aside seemingly mundane and vague projects like "Get Organized" because it isn't as fun as nearly every other aspect of your life and business. However, the stress lurking in the pile of laundry you haven't put away or the 187 emails you need to take action on is silently taking its toll on you right now, even if you are pretending to be unaware of it.

While I would never claim to be a neat freak for fear of being struck down by lightning, I do know that when life feels out of control my physical living space tends to follow suit. As a yogi, no doubt you have seen how your internal experience affects the external presentation you show the world. Spending time sorting and cleaning up helps me feel that some small part of my life is in order, even if much of it is in chaos.

One of my childhood friends would make a point of dressing up for school on days he was in a bad mood or on the verge of getting sick. He told me very simply that when he looks good he feels good. If he felt awful, he put extra effort into his appearance.

And guess what?

It elicited a positive response from others. Having people greet him and tell him that he looked nice was often enough to shake him out of his own head, because honestly it is hard to be grouchy while people are complimenting you.

While you may not be as interested in being complimented on your physical appearance, consider the following:

Have you ever practiced at a studio that was (ahem) less than cared for?

There's something about wiping dirt off your yoga mat - dirt your feet picked up from just walking across the floor - that is not only gross. It gives you the distinct experience that the environment is less than cared for, and a far cry from being sacred.

When you feel like a space (whether it is a home, studio or a temple) has been *thoughtfully* cared for however, it invites a certain spacious quality that can not only be moving, but can be the ground for inspired possibility. And you don't have to be a professional organizer to achieve this in your own world. All you need are a few of the basics, executed well.

Get Organized Now

Organized Living

Creating a living space you love turns your home into a true sanctuary and a place to rest and restore so you can be a better teacher. Spend 10-20 minutes each day decluttering one area of your living space. If you have more time, you can tackle an entire room, but it is best to start small because this can eat up your time quickly. Here's the technique:

1) Take four bags or bins labeled: Trash, Recycle, Donate, Belongs Elsewhere

2) In the area you are decluttering, place each item in one of those bags and put back anything that belongs where it is.

3) Immediately find the home of the "Belongs Elsewhere" items (seriously, do not wait on this one). You aren't finished until that bag is empty and everything is in its home.

4) Take out the trash and recycling so it isn't

cluttering your living space. Once the donation bag is full give it away to a local charity or a friend in need.

Organized Working

For most people, no matter what the organizational challenge at work is, sticking to your list or calendar will go a long way. Each time you sit down to take care of administration or plan a class or workshop, write out a list or add to your calendar the steps you need to take within the time frame you have. Do the most urgent or time-sensitive thing first and follow your list or scheduled time as best you can.

If you tend to procrastinate on priority items, they will be lurking in your mind while you work on everything you are doing to avoid them, sapping your creativity and peace of mind. Don't forget to leave an extra buffer of time to deal with important things that may come up. In short, stick to your calendar and your list and do first things first.

Organized Being

Meditation is a wonderful process for clearing mental clutter. If you have been practicing meditation for at least 20 minutes a day you may have had the experience of more grace, space or clarity *after* you meditate than before you sat down. If you are not a regular meditator, why not start now? Keep in mind that during meditation you don't need to force yourself to be clear or stop thinking.

Your job is to simply let go into the space that is already there underneath the mental clutter that may be temporarily covering it.

CHAPTER SIXTEEN

Productivity vs. Procrastination

When I sat down to write this chapter I turned on my computer ready to do some research, but while doing that I came across a funny video on Facebook. One video turned into four and then I found this neat website where you can learn how to make gourmet meals with just five ingredients. Then one of my friends asked if I wanted to meet her for tea so I did that and when I came home it was time to start making dinner so I promised I would get to it tomorrow - sound familiar yet?

Procrastination is such a cultural problem that it has been normalized under the weight of all the distractions we are surrounded by daily. We put off things that matter or tasks that move our lives forward in exchange for lofty promises that we will "do it later."

Procrastination goes arm in arm with poor organizational skills. Just think of any teacher you know whose classes chronically run overtime even with a rush job savasana.

Even if you don't procrastinate, chances are a lot of your students do. Letting unfinished business pile up causes stress, plain and simple. Luckily, yoga can be a powerful antidote to procrastination and boost productivity since it helps to shake the cobwebs out of the body and trip the circuit of inertia (another good reason for a strong personal practice).

The funny thing about procrastination is that whatever you are putting off must get done at some point. Anyone with procrastination pathology knows that waiting on an unfinished task creates more frustration that just doing things right away.

Maybe you have a traumatic memory or recurring nightmare of a scenario similar to this:

One of your high school teachers announces a major paper that is worth 40% of your grade and is due next month. The deadline slowly approaches, but there are more interesting things happening in your social circle and with your extracurriculars. Suddenly, it is the weekend of your best friend's birthday and your teacher reminds you that this major paper is due first thing Monday morning. Guess what? You haven't even begun the research needed for this mammoth project.

Oh the teen angst!

If you miss the birthday party your best friend will hate you forever and you will never get a date with the heartthrob you have had your eye on. If you don't write the paper, you will fail the class, be held back and your parents will disown you. You will never get into the school you wanted to go to. Your life is ruined. Right then and there, you promise yourself you will never be in this situation ever again. Dramatic? Yes. But everyone can probably relate to a do or die moment where they vowed to never put off something important ever again.

And yet, the pathological procrastinator will

illogically find themselves in some level of this situation over and over again, letting people down and hurting themselves. Procrastination means you exert the both the effort needed to get the job done in the first place *plus* the energy it takes to process the cortisol that is flooding your system. Enough studies have been done that we know this stress hormone negatively affects long term health and the capacity for stress management.

Exercise: Beat Procrastination Through Productivity

Productivity has become an entire industry in recent years with ingenious books, apps and sites devoted to the topic. One of the methods I use to overcome procrastination and increase productivity is inspired by Tim Ferriss, author of several books including my favourite, The 4 Hour Work Week.

Here is my spin on an exercise originally found on his blog (check out the digital resource package at the end of the book for more):

1) Start your morning with a yoga and/or meditation practice followed by a great breakfast.

2) Before looking at your emails or your phone, take a seat and jot down 3 or 4 "to-dos" that are causing you the most stress.

3) For each item ask yourself, "If I complete this

one thing today, will I feel a deep sense of accomplishment?"

4) Next ask yourself, "If I complete this one thing today, will it make my life easier, happier, or less cluttered?"

5) Last question. "Is someone counting on me to to complete this today who will be let down if I don't?"

6) Pick the "to-dos" that you answered "Yes" to most often. If you have an even number of affirmatives, pick the one that will lift the greatest burden off of you.

7) Block out a solid amount of time in your day to complete your chosen item. During that time, ignore distractions and get to work.

CHAPTER SEVENTEEN

Q is for Quit

In the past few chapters we have been exploring lessons around how to be more organized and productive. It may come as a shock, but quitting has personally saved me from wasting effort and made me a more successful person.

A few years ago, I attended a conference where one of the keynote speakers, <u>Arianna Huffington,</u> charted her journey to success. She had a major insight that forced her to change her relationship to work due to dangerous fatigue and burnout.

During her talk, she implored the audience to create some hard and fast rules around our health and self-care. For better quality sleep, she insisted a total purge of electronics in the bedroom. For a healthier relationship to our professional life, she insisted no more peeking at work related email after hours or on the weekend. As a yoga teacher this resonates with the message we deliver to our students and the way we promote well-being.

My favourite part of the talk however, was when she pointed out that the quickest way to get a shorter "to-do" list is to quit doing the things that aren't moving your life forward or that you simply do not enjoy. It reminded me that life is short and that there is too much good in the world to waste time on things that aren't feeding your soul.

Finishing something for the sake of finishing it is not a good use of your time when you are running a business. Since you wear so many hats as a teacher and business owner, being smarter about what you say "yes" to is a skill you must develop. However, there are times when you say "yes" to something only to find out it isn't going in the direction you had hoped.

For instance, if you teach at a studio that involves a forty-five minute commute and the class is consistently slow for more than a few months, it might make sense to quit teaching that class. Instead of teaching during that time what could you be doing with that extra three hours a week to move your business forward?

Quitting in this intelligent way isn't limited to business related items. Do you need to finish a book or movie you are lukewarm about? No. **Your leisure time is sacred and should be full of things that are deeply enjoyable and nourishing**.

At the beginning of this book, I asked you to think about your direction as a teacher and business owner. Although it may seem strange, quitting is in fact a champion of directionality because the energy you save from firmly closing the door on a loose end allows you to redistribute it to something that matters more.

Quitting also means that those loose items aren't floating around in your consciousness causing low grade anxiety. The next page is one of the most important in this book. You may wish to print it out and place somewhere in your home or office you frequently visit.

Quitting Checklist

Quit when...

You don't want it

You don't enjoy it

You no longer need it

It isn't helping

It isn't working even after you have tried many

angles

It isn't making you healthy

It is draining you constantly

CHAPTER SEVENTEEN

R is for Restore

One of the universal themes woven into most forms of physical asana deals with how high-level yoga cultivates energy rather than depletes it. The practice of restoration is easy to spot each time you guide students into savasana. In this sacred transition, you provide your students with the time and space to integrate all of the effort they have exerted throughout class.

It also reminds them how good it feels simply to do nothing in a relaxed state of pure contentment. In order to deliver a powerful experience as a teacher, however, it is important that you are no stranger to restoration in your own life.

Some teachers have this practice down pat: they take regular days off each week, eat healthy, nourishing food and are exemplars of self-care.

If, however, you land on the other end of the spectrum, you probably talk a good game but don't practice what you preach. While your students may never know just how undernourished you are as a teacher, your impact is the greatest when students feel your authenticity, a presence of being earned by backing up the advice you give with your own life.

Burnout

When teachers quit teaching for good, it isn't because they have seen and done it all and are ready for the next big challenge life has to offer.

Yoga teachers quit because they become disillusioned with the yoga industry and crash under the demands of a weekendless schedule with clients who feel the license to call for classes at all times.

The trouble is that as a yoga teacher, you are probably a natural giver, designed to go above and beyond the expectations of your clients. While this is an asset that assists you in delighting students, when mixed with the never ending pile of work responsibilities a business owner must confront, taking restoration seriously may be twice as challenging.

It is safe to assume that because you are reading this book you are motivated and interested in learning how to create a successful business, which means you are more likely to work longer and harder than the average yoga teacher. Your impressive work ethic is what will help you get things done, but you also need to make sure you have the downtime to let your brilliant business ideas arise. My most inspired ideas strike while in the sauna, during bodywork sessions or, you guessed it, during a yoga class.

Guard your downtime with the utmost rigidity and be strict with yourself and others about what this means. It may seem counterintuitive to think that consciously taking time away from your business could somehow be one of the keys to success, but as a yoga teacher, you know it is true since it is part of our culture and how we teach.

How to Restore your Body and Soul

Below are some ideas for soul and body restoration. Test drive a few and find out how restoring can make you more successful.

Take 2 days off per week (1 must be completely work free: no emails or returning phone calls).

Make sure your "work" is done by 9pm at the very latest each night.

Go on a retreat where you are the student not the teacher.

Read a non-yoga, non-business book, just for fun.

Spend an afternoon with your friends and promise not to speak about your classes, students or any aspect of work.

Get some bodywork (your job is physical so make a regular tune-up part of your routine).

Plan a fun day; go for a hike or to the beach, or to a sports event with someone you love to connect with.

Leave time and space in your personal yoga practice to restore. Practicing a daily savasana for at least 10 minutes will give you an experiential reminder of the power of letting go so you never ever skimp on it when you teach.

Practice Restorative yoga. Even if it is only once a month, attend a gentle or restorative class with a fabulous teacher. Allow yourself to be held by the powerful space they create rather than trying to do this in a self-led way.

Meditate daily.

CHAPTER EIGHTEEN

S is for Sales

"Sales", another word yogis traditionally shun. Let's first be clear, there is nothing wrong with giving something away for free. I have given thousands of dollars worth of content, classes and coaching away by donation or without any intent to ever be compensated. Personally, teaching yoga at women's shelters, for people dealing with cancer and youth at risk has provided the most spiritually potent moments of my career.

There is however a shadow in the yoga world around sales and the exchange of money. Having observed the evolution of hundreds of teachers, I have seen an emergence of a smug superiority in the faction of people who feel that yoga should be free for all and that teachers and studios have no right to charge more than the most modest fee for their classes. These teachers are typically part-timers and feel that they are teaching for the love of yoga only. As mentioned above, there absolutely are populations that will benefit from free classes, and anyone who can serve them should do so when possible. These classes are not what I am speaking of. The problem I have with the "free for everyone" mentality is that it robs a professional teacher of a sustainable livelihood.

Amateurs vs. Pros

Consider this idea from Steven Pressfield's book "The War of Art" (a must read):

"*The conventional interpretation is that the amateur pursues his calling out of love, while the pro does it for money. Not the way I see it. In my view, the amateur does not love the game enough. If he did he would not pursue it as a sideline, distinct from his "real" vocation. The professional loves it so much he dedicates his life to it. He commits full-time.*"

No yoga teacher gets into teaching for fame and fortune (if you did, you picked the wrong career).

However, there is no reason you can't have a perfectly comfortable and enjoyable lifestyle full of opportunities.

You may not like it, but in order to be successful, you must learn how to be a sales person. You need not be sleazy or cheesy to do it, but at the end of the day, what you earn depends on how effectively you deliver what your students and clients want with a price tag you both feel comfortable with.

How to Be an Awesome, Authentic Salesperson

1) Get comfortable with what you are charging.

If you are fresh out of yoga teacher training you probably don't have the chops and expertise to charge a hundred dollars an hour for a private class. However, if you need to drive for more than half an hour both ways or the class is at a busy time of day, it might make sense.

2) Believe in the product.

As a yoga teacher, selling your classes and workshops should in theory be a breeze, because you know first-hand how powerful yoga has been for you. Yet most teachers aren't natural self-promoters. Just like yoga, regular practice is the way to go. Review the chapter on marketing as often as you need to.

3) Understand the needs of your clients.

In the chapter on how to identify your ideal client, we also dove into understanding what your students want and need. Speak to those same needs when you are offering your workshop or class.

4) Understand the "Pain Points" of your clients.

Knowing what your clients want and need is very important to the sales process. Of equal importance is understanding the unique problems they have. If your ideal client is a high level executive with a stressful job, their personal pain point will be different than a retired person who is dealing with back pain. Just as you might customize your class differently for these two students, you should also customize your pitch and what you offer.

5) Be a specialist.

While you may be excited to share the wide-ranging benefits of yoga, remember who you are talking to, what they need and what their pain points are. Highlight your experience in those areas instead of overwhelming your clients with too much information that doesn't relate to them.

CHAPTER TWENTY

T is for Time

Time is Money.

We have heard that a million times before - usually from our friends in more traditional careers - but have you considered the true value of your time?

Maybe you have already noticed it happening, but as you build relationships with your community, students and other instructors will begin to pull you aside to talk after class for a few minutes or email you questions.

My personal boundary on this has evolved. If someone asks me a yoga-related question that I can answer in under five minutes and I have the time to do so, I will. If, however I get a long list of questions or the matter deserves more time, I will suggest that the person book a private session or a coaching call with me.

Obviously some situations require a donation of time and effort. For instance, if you know someone is struggling financially and they need a bit of help, you could offer some of your time if you have it to spare.

However, I would advise ensuring you aren't being taken advantage of, remembering that, at worst, some people will feel entitled to use your generous heart and, at best, they simply don't have their financial priorities straight. I have heard people bemoan their financial situation fishing for a freebie with a five dollar latte in one hand and purse worth more than my monthly rent in the other.

Dealing with Time-Consuming Questions

My preferred way to deal with an in-depth yoga question is to say:

 "We can work on it in class because it will take a bit of time, so just remind me next week before we begin and I will get to it".

This one sentence has helped me build a beautiful rapport with students as they tend to return and ask the question again. In this instance everyone wins. The returning student is financially benefiting the studio, the other students win by getting new information and the student feels special to get a little bit of extra attention and care.

If the issue is surrounding an injury or more urgent question, the next step would be to suggest a private session. If you are teaching at a studio, always check what their policy is surrounding this. Respect the fact that if the studio has done the work to bring students in they may require you to work with that student in their space as per your teaching agreement. There are additional liabilities to consider if you take a student out of the studio into a private setting, so it is best to avoid any conflict with the studio or the student and be clear about the expectations and agreement upfront.

Overall, it is important to assess how much "free" time you are giving away and attach appropriate value to your services, which allows you to be a true professional. Along with the exercise of "empowered evaluation" from earlier in the book, complete this time assessment so you can get a handle on your time for money.

Time and Energy Audit

Money can be made and lost, but you'll never get your time back.

1) Pick one class that you're feeling a bit drained or uneasy about.

2) Write down the length of the class.

3) Add the travel time to and from.

4) Add the length of any "awkward pockets" between that class and the next one your have scheduled; you know what I'm talking about, those time slots that are too long to be ignored, but too short to get anything meaningful accomplished (including relaxing).

5) Add in any preparation or follow-up time required for the class.

6) Write down any energy leaks within the class - is the style not one you click with, are there

students who are high-maintenance or disrespectful, is the class size uncomfortable (either too big or too small), do you feel supported by the studio or the client, are you fairly compensated, etc.?

7) How is the timing of the class? Is it earlier in the morning or later at night than you can comfortably accommodate?

If this is a gray area or if you're having trouble figuring out how much your time is worth, try this simple equation: add up your time and hours spent on this class per week, then divide it by the pay you receive, and see if that number feels like a fair per-hour rate for you (Hours / Pay = Your Current Rate).

All of these factors contribute to what you should be charging for a class. After writing them all down, how do you feel about the payment you are receiving for it? Is it fair, given the true cost to you (i.e. your business) as discovered in this exercise?

If it is less than what you need, consider

increasing your rates. I have created a few strategies on how to do this in the resource section.

CHAPTER TWENTY-ONE

U is for Unite

Remember our lesson on joining together as teachers?

I asked you to start teaming up with like minded instructors to support one another. If you haven't taken the "Share the Love" challenge yet, I hope you will be inspired to do it after reading this chapter.

Have you ever celebrated a big success and thought about what started it all?

For most people, it was a few words of encouragement from a trusted mentor or conversation with a loved one that sparked something inside of them. That spark, no matter how small, is enough to set you off on a path to creating something you hadn't dreamt was possible before. A little bit of support goes a long way and the road to success depends upon it over and over again.

Sadly, in the last decade I have witnessed disconcerting things happen between yoga instructors time and time again. The first rude "unyogic" awakening I received came after helping another teacher who was very ill by subbing her class. At the time, I was a new instructor without a weekly class and the teacher I stepped in for had a steady footing with one of the bigger studios in the city we lived in. The class went well and many of the students made a point to thank me afterwards. Several asked when I would have a class of my own at the studio. Needless to say, I was thrilled.

I emailed the teacher a few days later to see how she was feeling and to let her know I would gladly sub her class anytime. Her response floored me. Rather than thank me for stepping in last minute, she said she would not be contacting me again to sub. Her "advice" was to make sure I didn't teach a strong class when subbing for another teacher, should I ever be given the opportunity.

Once I picked my jaw up off the floor I reached out to a friend of mine who worked at the studio as an administrator. My friend told me that there had been so much positive feedback about my class that it threatened the regular teacher. My friend nonchalantly continued:

"Don't take it personally though, it happens all the time. Most yoga teachers talk a good game, but they don't treat one another well."

After I moved to a smaller city the situation changed, but I never forgot that experience or how much of a makeover our industry needs.

While you shouldn't waste time on people that are clearly only out for themselves, remember that when you encounter a teacher who seems stingy, protective or cynical that you have an opportunity to evolve our profession and find a healthier response to the perceived competition.

Uniting with Other Teachers

My strategy in relationship to other teachers has been to proactively eliminate any sense of greed or competition. I routinely promote classes and events other teachers are hosting whenever they land in my class. If a teacher moves to my hometown, I make as many introductions to studios and students looking for private classes as possible.

Closed door teaching communities are widespread and their karma is very deep so I have made it a personal mission to change the standard.

If you do no other exercise from this book, I urge you to become a connector in your own yoga community. To those of you who don't directly see how this will help your personal success, I assure you, your own generosity will gain you the friendship, support and respect of other teachers. If you ever find yourself in need of a new class or help promoting your own events, the same teachers you cared for will be by your side.

Here are some ideas to help you cultivate a stronger, more positive community with teachers so you can cheer each other on towards success.

Share an event, class or simple expression of respect and care for another instructor publicly with your fans on social media.

Shower another teacher with authentic praise for their hard work and dedication to their practice and students.

If another instructor comes to your class, let everyone know about their upcoming workshop.

Offer to collaborate on a project or specialty workshop with someone you respect.

Spend time talking about the ups and downs of this profession with a group of instructors.

Find ways to help each other through the rough patches.

Recognizing that we are all one is the very foundation that yoga was built on. It is time for teachers to unite authentically and share this beautiful and rich path together.

CHAPTER TWENTY-TWO

V is for Value

When you hear the word *"value"* what do you think of?

The discount super store?

Bargain basement prices?

Or do you think of value as getting something more than you originally expected?

As teachers, value is an important theme that affects far more than what you charge versus what you offer. Some facets of value also dictate how worthy you feel as an instructor.

To begin, write down your thoughts on the following:

1) Do you feel valued by the clients, students and studios you work with?

2) Do you value yourself appropriately?

3) Does teaching yoga the way that you do provide value to the people you work with?

4) What could you do to offer even more to the people you work with and increase your value?

How to Provide Value

Be Professional
You could be the world's most knowledgeable teacher, but if you are a hot mess when it comes to arriving at your classes on time or interact irresponsibly with students, you will become more trouble than you are worth. Unprofessional teachers work against their own value, so tidy up any unkempt behaviour as quickly and cleanly as possible.

Be Consistent
While this is also an aspect of being professional, success depends on offering serious value consistently as a yoga teacher. A consistent tone, energy level and class level all give your students somewhere to plant their feet while they work to expand in their practice. Being the solid, trustworthy lodestone in a yoga class allows your students the freedom to explore the jungle of their body and inner experience knowing their guide is right beside them. On a practical level, staying consistent with what you

promised to offer in the class is important.

Imagine if you went to the dentist and he or she checked your vision instead, you would not walk away feeling like you got what you signed up for.

Yet you may have been to yoga classes where the teacher announces "Hi everyone, let's do something different today."

Learning new things is never bad, and certainly there are times when the situation may allow a bit of leeway such as a one-on-one private class. However, it is important to remember that the class does not exist to entertain you. If you are "switching it up" because you feel bored, consider that you may have temporarily lost sight of what you have agreed to deliver.

Your classes need to evolve as you continue to learn and grow, but if you are scheduled to teach a weekly Restorative class and lead a Power Flow instead, you aren't giving your students what they asked for (and paid for).

Be Unique

The fun part of adding value to the service of teaching is that you can decide what that looks like. Continuing education in your field of interest as an instructor is an amazing way to deliver a unique and therefore valuable experience to your students. My interest in Chinese medicine led me to become an acupuncturist and infuse that philosophy into yoga, creating a special brand of Yin Yang practice that I now train other instructors to teach. One of my good friends dove deeply into anatomy and functional movement and became the local expert in their hometown.

If you truly embrace this principle you will unlock one to the keys to success: **You can never be in competition with another teacher or studio if you are sharing your unique take on yoga and the wisdom you have learned.**

Even if you teach the exact same style as the instructor down the street, you are both delivering your flavor and expression of that practice.

Value Booster Exercise

In many of the exercises so far we have spent time and energy working on things for the future and tidying up loose ends. Of equal importance is the act of celebrating your own worth. The road to success need not be a constant struggle trying to get somewhere into the future.

Success comes in many forms. It is present in the gratitude of your students as much as it is in the dollars you have in the bank. Both reflect to you that you are doing a good job and are respected by the people you work with and we need both types of success. We need to be paid a sustainable wage that supports our growth and fuels our lifestyle *and* we need positive feedback from our students and studio owners.

Begin to boost the value of your classes. Brainstorm ways that feel authentic to you and your style.

Do you give a brief head massage to your students before they let go in Savasana?

Do you follow up with emails each week or create a home program for them to follow? Are you taking a new training to add to the knowledge you provide in class?

A true professional knows that adding value does not mean discounting your rates but instead offering more so that you can eventually increase your rates in a way that sustains them while the client continues to feels like they are getting more than they pay for.

Next, honour the ways in which others value you. I keep a collection of the notes of praise or thanks I have been given over the years. When I doubt who I am as a teacher, these letters and gifts lift me out of my funk and never fail to humble and inspire me to do whatever I can to help more people. This collection also reminds me to advocate for my own worth when I negotiate rates with new clients and studios. I highly suggest you start a collection of your own. While some might view this as egotistical, you will probably find as I have that it is a constant reminder to show up and give your students all that you have.

CHAPTER TWENTY-THREE

W is for Workshop

Throughout the course of this book I have given you some important exercises, insights and contemplations to help you become a more successful yoga teacher. This chapter is no different because it deals with something that is crucial to developing your unique contribution to the yoga world and, if done just right, is a huge part of financial success.

Teaching workshops sets you apart from the crowd and simultaneously allows you to follow your deepest passion as a teacher. It is a labour of love to research and prepare valuable content for your students. This process, while time-consuming, is worth the effort--especially when you consider that a solid workshop pays much more than a "one-off" private or public yoga class.

From Workshop Shy to Workshop Savvy

Creating a successful workshop is so much more than just slapping a poster on the wall and hoping for the best. You must create something that is inviting enough to have your students set aside the time and money to attend. To get started, focus on the following areas:

Powerful Content

In order to host a successful workshop, pick a topic your Ideal Client cares about. Once you decide, it's time to break down your core message into the key points the workshop will focus upon and how you will present each one. Remember, the session must focus on what your students really want. If you are interested in teaching a workshop about yoga for athletes, ask local athletes what would appeal to them.

Should you focus on their pain points or on peak performance?

Workshop Planner Sample

Topic: Yoga for Athletes

Main Points:
1. Improve Performance
2. Prevent Injuries
3. Reduce Recovery Time
4. Stay Calm and Focused

Main Take Away: A 20-minute yoga routine they can practice during their training

Marketing Plan:
1. Set up weekly emails to send to targeted segment of current student base.
2. Pre-schedule social media blasts regarding the event 2-3 times/ week.
3. Reach out to local studios, gyms and other spots your Ideal Client might frequent.
4. Create beautiful visuals on your website or event page.

What will be the take-aways of the workshop?

Powerful Promo

To make sure the room is packed, you need to utilize a good marketing strategy. This need not be complex or expensive, but it must be effective. If you are going to host the workshop with a studio, create an agreed-upon time-line for your social media and email blasts. If you are doing it all on your own, start early. Trying to put a workshop together with less than six weeks of lead time can be very challenging unless you have a team of people helping you. To get started, write a series of emails and social media posts that you can schedule to go out at regular intervals rather than writing them on the fly.

Powerful Experience

Once the date arrives and the room is full and ready to learn from you, how do you actually deliver a great workshop?

Most teachers find the workshop experience

much more daunting than teaching a regular class because the stakes are higher and there is more time to fill. Creating a great vibe means moving beyond your jitters and progressing through the workshop with confidence. Make sure you hit the points you promised to make in your promotional material and respond to the interest in the room. How you structure your time will depend on your style, but as long as you make space to express your point, work on it through practice it together, and answer any questions that arise, you'll have enough to get started.

As a side note, no matter how well you plan your workshop, there's always going to be somebody who will pull focus from the main points or ask questions that get you off-topic. My biggest workshop fail was when I gave valuable amounts of time to off-topic questions or unrelated topics and missed the major point of the workshop.

How to deal with this is to let those enthusiastic people know that you can come back to their question if there is still time at the end. This gives you a chance to approach them afterwards, and perhaps offer a one-on-one session. One of my best clients started out with a question during a workshop about chanting. I spoke with her afterwards and suggested she book a private session, which led to years of well-paid and very rewarding classes with her.

CHAPTER TWENTY-FOUR

X is for XXX

Now that I've got your attention, let's talk about sex and teaching. In fact, let's talk about all of the ethical boundaries around teaching yoga. As an instructor you have a responsibility to your students to be professional and not manipulate their vulnerability. We all know that loose boundaries and inappropriate behavior have been the downfall of more than one yoga teacher and yet few people speak openly about this big topic. Let's begin to scratch the surface and figure out where you stand.

Sex

It is so common for a rockstar teacher's career to go down in flames due to a sexual scandal that it no longer shocks anyone when they hear that yet *another* spiritual guru was caught in bed with a student.

Personally, I have a strict "no dating students" policy, and for good reason. All but two of the dozens of such teacher/student unions I have witnessed in the last 10 years were short-lived and in a word: disastrous.

The whole thing is very tricky. Teachers are easily put on a pedestal and given power by their students. It makes sense that when a student falls in love with the practice, they may also develop feelings for the person introducing them to this new and wonderful world. As an instructor, it is beautiful to see people infatuated with yoga when you have devoted so much of your life to it. That alone creates a sweet bond with regular students.

Occasionally that bond will be taken to the next level. While it can be very flattering to be approached romantically by a wide-eyed student who thinks the world of you (ignoring the fact that they only see you at work and have no idea who you are the other 23 hours of the day), there is a skewed power dynamic in place, which is not a healthy foundation for a relationship.

It can hurt your reputation big time if you are known as a teacher who routinely dates students. A teacher who is trolling probably isn't paying attention to anything outside of their libido's limited sphere of awareness. This will affect the safety of the students if said instructor is not looking out for their well-being but is distracted by other motives instead.

Giving Medical or Personal Advice

You know that your students feel connected to you and that your class is a major catalyst for them to get healthy or feel more positive. So it is natural that you might be the first person they turn to when they are about to make a major life decision. It is also understandable for someone to think that because you know so much about yoga, you might also be aware of effective supplements or have dietary recommendations to share.

If you have ever been put in this position you know how tricky it can be to navigate. On one hand you will feel genuinely compelled to give your advice from the nurturing place within you. On the other hand you are probably giving uninformed advice. I don't mean to burst anyone's bubble, but yoga teachers are not health care professionals (unless you are actually a doctor, nutritionist, etc., in which case you are well aware you can't give medical advice legally unless you are wearing that hat).

Personal advice can be even more murky. I would be very cautious about doling out any definitive advice that could have major implications on anyone's life. Instead, try offering supportive strategies or suggesting a great practitioner to work through the issue more in-depth.

Trust me when I say that if you begin to give major non-yoga related advice, you open yourself to becoming a crutch for people. This leads to a lot of weird interpersonal issues (including being blamed if something goes wrong).

The Problem with Listening to Your Body

We've just outlined how to avoid overstepping your position as a yoga teacher. Ironically, while many teachers cross interpersonal boundaries, when it comes to the actual class and the job we're being paid to do, most teachers aren't present enough. Let me explain using one of the most commonly abused phrases in the studio:

"Listen to your body" or "Do what feels right."

These sweet phrases *sound* like we're giving our students permission to take care of themselves and find their own way during the practice. However, it is high time we examined these well-intentioned standards thoughtfully. I would be so bold as to say that most teachers that utter these words are just repeating something that they themselves have heard a thousand times. At best, "listen to your body" is a throw-away line used to fill space. At worst, these instructions can lead to chaos and even injury.

Defense

On the part of the teacher, these words are often a casually defensive move. For some teachers, the use of "do what feels right"-type phrases comes in response to dogmatic schools of yoga and the guru model. We also know that postmodern people don't like being told what to do in a definitive manner, so it makes sense that as teachers we have modeled a language that *suggests* rather than *instructs*. In fact, some teachers have such a hard time with "instruction" that they refer to themselves as guides and not teachers.

In other cases, the person leading the class is using "listen to your body" as a blanket disclaimer that absolves them personally from being responsible for the class. You run the risk of becoming a disconnected teacher if you have a habit of using a disclaimer in lieu of actually observing the room and helping students as needed.

Confidence Issues

Another big reason for throwing in a routine "do

what feels best" is lack of self-confidence. Rather than openly telling students what to do, you leave them with half a dozen options that confuse and distract. The problem isn't with giving your students options if they need them. The problem is when you are giving vague instructions because you are uncomfortable being clear and definitive.

Most teachers, especially new ones, identify this as a felt sense of lacking the knowledge to lead the sequence. On one hand, you shouldn't teach what you don't know. But you should also consider that you might actually know more than you think. Continuing education and practice will help you to build self-confidence over time.

Doing What Feels Right Isn't Always Best

"Do what feels right" as a statement may seem like a small thing and you could call me picky for addressing it, but here is why I think it is so important: the unexamined overuse of such a phrase is going to land your students squarely in their comfort zone. If someone tends to push themselves too hard, then the most extreme version of the pose will "feel right." If they tend to stop at the first bead of sweat, they will listen to the status quo and follow that as the truth of "what they need in this moment."

When I go to class it is to be guided and to learn. If I truly listened to my body, I would probably stay home and eat a donut. When your students make the effort to show up to your class, they are showing up to listen, learn, trust and inquire.

Staying loosey-goosey in the face of the enormous honour your students pay you by showing up reminds me of something my friend Jeff Carreira once said to me: a teacher who doesn't carry the power and respect they are being paid is like someone who is armed with an Uzi pretending it is a pea shooter. Everyone knows what you are packing and yet you are undermining and downplaying the authority and knowledge you have. In short, probing these particular phrases will help you determine if you are really using them to help create space, or if you are inadvertently letting your students off the hook from their own unfolding.

If you are considering dropping these familiar phrases from your vocabulary, what can you do to allow for space and options without being overly casual?

1) At the beginning of class, take a moment to explain the difference between pain and discomfort, and let students know that if they need additional modifications to ask you for help during the class.

2) Ask if anyone has injuries or special considerations before the class begins.

3) Welcome a rest pose which you demonstrate before the class starts (show one option, not five) and remind the class of that option once during the class.

4) If you do feel the need to fill space with the phrase "do what you want," instead, try being silent and looking very closely to see who might need a different direction.

CHAPTER TWENTY-FIVE
Y is for Yes

Several times during the course of this book, I have made the statement that success depends on saying "no" to the right things in order to make the space and time you need to focus on your next steps. In this chapter, let's think about what it takes to say "yes" as well.

The Nature of Yes

In a moment of inspiration or excitement you decided to say YES to becoming a yoga teacher. In the chapter on aspiration, I asked you to connect with the original energy that made you embark on this journey. An authentic "yes" is the moment you decide to take action and realize your hopes and dreams. You seal that intention with a wholehearted commitment to venture forward, often into uncharted territory.

When you say yes you are devoting yourself to something without knowing where the

promise will lead you or how it will turn out.

Saying yes is for the risk taker who is willing to put hard work, love and soul into something knowing full well that it may not turn out the way they had planned. In the moments when a whole-hearted affirmative erupts from within you, it doesn't feel like a choice, it feels like a force.

Connecting to Yes
On the road to success, you quickly learn that there are periods of time where you feel the burden of "yes" as well. It may seem that the energetic current that moved you has suddenly evaporated and you begin to wonder if it was ever there in the first place, or if it was simply a wild figment of your imagination. These moments are gut-wrenching and can send you into a spiral. When this happens try one of these tactics to reconnect with your original positivity.

Seek out a friend on the path
There is absolutely nothing that gets me fired up about teaching and creating resources for my fans and clients the way a good collaboration

does. Even something as simple as spending devoted time speaking about your dreams or troubleshooting the things that aren't working are key if you intend to succeed in a big way. As a teacher, so much of your work is self-generated so why not share that challenge with someone who can relate. Collaboration and building friendships among peers is a beautiful way to amplify your output and rekindle "yes."

Teach
Spending time with people who love you and believe in you is one way to boost confidence in moments of self-doubt, but when it comes to connecting with "yes" the best remedy is sometimes to teach! Putting attention on the practice you love and the career you have given so much to is a great way to break through confusion and reconnect with why you are here in the first place.

Take time off
One of the best things to do if you are feeling low-energy and uninspired is to rest. It may seems obvious, but most people avoid taking

time off when work feels like a burden. Many yoga teachers feel guilty about subbing out the odd class if they are feeling down and out but not stricken with any illness. While it is important to be professional and not flaky when it comes to looking after your classes, ask yourself if you can truly deliver the session your students deserve in those moments. If possible, don't let your battery get low. Instead of burning out and needing sporadic days to regroup, build real days off into your schedule as well as regular retreats and self-care.

Finally, remember to think carefully about what you are saying "yes" to on the small scale. It is better to do a few things well with your energy than spread yourself thin or be pulled in twenty directions. Staying focused will help make everything you take on an expression of that original, authentic "yes."

CHAPTER TWENTY-SIX

Z is for Zone

What is your teaching zone?

Do you have a special niche or framework that you want to focus upon?

Finding and developing your zone is essential to success and might be one of the most difficult lessons of all for yoga teachers. If you are anything like me, you love yoga because there is so much to learn. One could spend lifetimes learning the different practices and philosophies that we put under the umbrella called yoga. While I would never want to deter you from following whatever your educational interests may be, I do want you to think about narrowing your field and getting into your zone in order to achieve success.

When I began teaching, I wanted to teach as many styles of yoga as possible. The more I learned the more I wanted to expand. In theory, I believed that students would rather have a teacher who could lead them through a handful of styles. Yet when I looked for a class, I gravitated towards people who had steeped themselves in a certain tradition. What's interesting is I wanted to be a diverse teacher for my students, but I wanted a teacher who specialized in one area for myself. I spent a lot of time spreading out my education and while it was wonderful, as I began trying to build a business my message was vague.

What I found was that I was vying for clients in a soup full of teachers who could all also teach 10 styles of yoga. I didn't have a defined bubble that was unique and because of that, it took a number of years for my ideal clients to find me. Once I realized that "less is more" I stopped trying to be all things to all people and started focusing on my personal brand of Yin Yang Yoga. Once the zone was defined I was able to emerge from the generic soup and focus my attention on fine-tuning my chops, learning more and evolving my teaching.

Find and Develop your Zone

Your zone is the area of your teaching that has its own particular quality and purpose. To help you define and move into your zone, work through the following exercise.

1) What does your ideal client want?

Does your ideal client prefer a particular style and a teacher who is very knowledgeable in that area, or do they want someone who can mix it up?

Do they want a teacher who sticks to a similar focus like functional anatomy or a spiritual theme, or do they want someone who regularly changes their approach?

2) What special interest in yoga do you have in common with your Ideal Client?

How can that shared interest become a unique offering?

3) Is there any further education (courses, reading material, a coach or a well-versed teacher) that can help you get into the zone?

4) How can you share and bring students into your zone (blog, special workshops, conferences)?

At first, it may feel suffocating to even contemplate narrowing your expression of yoga into just one zone. It certainly did for me. However, remember you don't need to limit yourself or your knowledge. Finding and developing your zone is a way of clarifying your message and highlighting a part of your yoga education that you and your ideal clients are interested in.

Clarity is a beautiful thing that helps people connect with you. Be creative and if you find after a good length of time and authentic effort you want to change course, you will know how to discover your next zone.

Closing Thoughts

Being a Successful Yoga Teacher will mean different things to different people. Your definition of success may be a prospering studio or a high-end client base. You may wish to travel and teach all over the world, or you might dream of planting your roots and growing a tight-knit yoga community. However, I doubt that success to you looks like struggling to make ends meet or resenting and eventually abandoning the practice you felt compelled to teach. It may not always seem to be this way, but your success is in your hands. It is time for yoga teachers to stop waiting for full classes and well-paying clients to fall into their laps. We need now, more than ever, to start being creative about how we share our knowledge with the world.
The world doesn't need anymore cynical, stressed-out and run down people.

It needs your strength and spirit, your compassion and interest to be amplified.

You can't teach if you can't eat.

So if you are physically, emotionally or spiritually hungry, let all of these ideas be your food.

Take them seriously.

Take yourself seriously and create the success you are looking for.

To your happiness and growth,

Erin Aquin
www.aquinyoga.com

To access your exclusive bonus resource package including downloadable worksheets, videos, inspirational articles and tips, visit: www.aquinyoga.com/az-resources

About the Author

Erin Aquin is an International Yoga Teacher born and raised in Hamilton, Ontario. With over a decade of teaching experience, Erin is a passionate yogi and a powerful, unapologetic public speaker who believes that yoga teachers must take on their business approach as a spiritual and self-worth practice. Through coaching, workshops, teacher training programs and her popular blog on www.aquinyoga.com, Erin reaches thousands of Yoga teachers and students monthly to help them thrive on the mat and in their lives. Currently she lives in Boston with her partner when she isn't traveling to work with teachers and studios or leading her 200 hour Correspondence Yin Yang Teacher Training Program. When not teaching and writing, Erin enjoys hiking in warm climates, things made of chocolate, kittens and eating wonderful food with good company.

Made in the USA
Charleston, SC
16 January 2017